HEARING THINGS

Philip Osment

HEARING THINGS

OBERON BOOKS
LONDON

WWW.OBERONBOOKS.COM

First published in 2019 by Oberon Books Ltd
521 Caledonian Road, London N7 9RH
Tel: +44 (0) 20 7607 3637 / Fax: +44 (0) 20 7607 3629
e-mail: info@oberonbooks.com
www.oberonbooks.com

PB ISBN: 9781786827203
E ISBN: 9781786827197

Cover image: Arthur Bentley

Printed and bound by 4EDGE Limited, Hockley, Essex, UK.
eBook conversion by Lapiz Digital Services, India.

10 9 8 7 6 5 4 3 2 1

Introduction

Playing ON was set up in 2010 to give voice to disenfranchised people and to create professional theatre of the highest artistic quality. The company engages with the target group, running drama workshops and creating scratch performances. The aim is to translate these authentic voices into new theatre scripts that inspire audiences through an urgent and truthful portrayal of life in contemporary Britain. It is intended that, through taking part in Playing On workshops and shared performances, participants gain skills for life and are empowered to re-engage with education, training and employment.

Our first production focused on the lives of young fathers in prison. After a successful run at the Roundhouse in the autumn of 2010, the company took the decision to turn its attention to mental health service users and professionals. There followed five years of research and development that included work with a range of agencies and institutions, including residencies in locked psychiatric wards.

The company's process consists of creating characters and bringing these characters into relationship with each other to create improvised scenes and story, adopting and adapting techniques that Playing ON's CEO and co-artistic director Jim Pope and I had learnt in our work with the director Mike Alfreds.

The format usually involves a series of weekly or bi-weekly workshops with the participation of both staff and service users. This is followed by an intensive rehearsal process culminating in some kind of improvised performance.

In using lived experience to create fictional characters and stories, participants come to an appreciation of each other's skill and insights as people. It enhances self-esteem, diminishes stigma, and gives a sense of achievement which might have been missing from their lives for many years.

One tricky aspect of running workshops where both staff and patients are present is that the patients are wary of being assessed, which might affect perceptions of how well or ill they are. Staff might at the same time feel threatened by a lack of boundaries. However, the process can break down boundaries in a safe way. When we worked on a locked psychiatric ward at Homerton Univeristy Hospital we created scenes where patients played staff and staff played patients. The performance on another ward drew staff and patients together and the director of the unit commented on the value of her nurses seeing patients' accurate and humorous depictions of themselves. She felt it encouraged them to see the person and not just their diagnosis. One patient clearly felt liberated by the experience; he was heard to say, "I'm off to drama to be mad and it doesn't matter." In fact after our residency at the Maudsley Hospital, it was noted that participants were discharged because their recovery had been more rapid than expected. This was attributed to their attendance at the workshops.

At times over the five years of research and development, the company would also develop scratch performances using a combination of professional actors and service users. These were more developed pieces looking at relationships of staff and patients and situations thrown up by our residencies, crafted into something more resembling a play. These scratch performances were presented to audiences in theatres and hospitals.

By spring 2016 we had given a number of such performances and an application had been made to the Arts Council for a professional production that would be written by me. When this bid was successful, I was faced with the task of somehow bringing together all that research and all these performances to create a script. It was a rather daunting prospect.

One of my concerns was to avoid the pitfall of demonising the psychiatrist and falling into the rather easy trap of showing him or her as the villain of the piece. At the same time, the psychiatrist's role and the need at times to constrain people suffering from psychosis through sectioning creates a power imbalance which underpins what is often a combative relationship. This can result in patients finding themselves caught in double binds, as described in the play. If they express anger at being constrained against their will, or show lack of compliance with a drug regime because the medication has unpleasant side-effects, then this is seen to be proof that they are ill. However during the course of our research the psychiatrists we met were all too aware of these contradictions and were often trying to help the patients manage their symptoms and healing process. There is a push to develop the idea of co-production, where ex-patients are enlisted as advocates and peer mentors, whose lived experiences give them insights which can prove effective in aiding other patients' recovery.

The truth is that psychiatrists themselves are on their own journeys and have a whole range of approaches. Within psychiatry there is an ongoing debate about the use of talking therapies. The medical approach focuses on the idea of chemical imbalances in the brain which might arise because of genetic susceptibility, whereas the emphasis of psychologists would tend to be on trauma going back to childhood and its impact on the patient's wellbeing. But talking therapies are time-consuming. Lack of funding, time constraints, the need to see as many patients as possible and the need to free up beds all mean that medication is used as a first resort, because it guarantees a more speedy diminution of symptoms and therefore a more rapid discharge.

The medical model raises concerns about the whole process of diagnosis. Often patients find themselves classified differently depending on the observations and bias of the last psychiatrist they saw. These classifications themselves have been made in what could be seen as an arbitrary and subjective manner. In *Hearing Things*, I think Nicholas is all too aware of these contradictions, which makes it particularly difficult for him to contend with his father's characterisation of psychiatry as being non-scientific. It seemed to me that for the psychiatrist who sees the value of a more psychological approach, like Nicholas, this can prove challenging.[1] I wanted to show that he is also caught in a double bind, and explore how his well-intentioned treatment of Janet exposes him to possible litigation. I found online newspaper reports of similar incidents. This double bind means that he retreats into the role of entrenched expert and is overcautious about discharging Innocent.

These are some of the issues which led me to make my

---

1   For a fuller exploration of the anti-psychiatry argument see "Cracked: Why Psychiatry is Doing More Harm Than Good" by James Davies.

central character a psychiatrist who is having a mental breakdown. It was partly informed too, by experiences on the ward where it was sometimes difficult for us to distinguish staff from patients – in one instance, a staff member who was under pressure because of lack of space for our workshop, approached Jim and delivered a panicky monologue about the problem, which caused Jim to think at first that he was dealing with a patient. One psychiatrist observed to us that the patients do eventually leave the hospital; it is often the staff who become institutionalised.

The characters themselves are amalgams of people that we met during residencies and characters developed by the actors during rehearsals for the scratch performances. So, for instance, Janet is based on a character created by Jeanette Rourke, who plays her in our production. Jeanette also created an improvisation from research, of strategies for dealing with hearing voices which has been used in the play. There were numerous incarnations of Innocent based on work by Michael Amaning, an associate member of the company. I have made my own additions and adjustments and re-imaginings. The scene where Innocent reads the Marvin Gaye speech arose from my observation that sometimes patients who were still quite ill had a perspective on the character they had created; a perspective which they might lack with relation to their own experiences. However, this was a scene imagined and created in the writing process. It is interesting that audiences sometimes falsely assume that the script arises from verbatim material – something I take as a compliment.

Philip Osment
13 December 2018

Characters

NICHOLAS
46, a psychiatrist in a London hospital – also seen
at ages 10 and 20

PATRICK
Nicholas's father, a retired oncologist

JANET
a patient in a psychiatric hospital

GRACE
Nicholas's wife, a vicar

HOPE
a Ghanaian woman, a nurse

INNOCENT
20, Hope's son

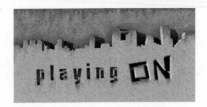

Playing ON is a theatre company and social enterprise set up in 2010 to produce quality theatre transforming the lives of disenfranchised people. The company exists to develop and promote theatre as a method for the powerless and the powerful to actively explore the key issues of a shared context. The company translates authentic voices and real life stories into high quality new writing. Through taking part in Playing ON workshops and performances, participants can engage with professional theatre, gain skills for life and are empowered to re-engage with education, training and employment.

Playing ON is led by Artistic Director Jim Pope.
Our patron is Mike Alfreds.

@PlayingON_

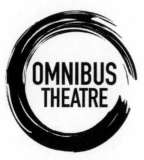

About Omnibus Theatre

Omnibus Theatre is a multi award-winning independent theatre in Clapham, South London. The Stage's Fringe Theatre of the Year 2019 nominee, recipient of the Peter Brook/Royal Court Theatre Support Award 2016 and Offie winner 2017. The heart of our ambitious programme, inspired by our building's literary heritage, lies in both classics re-imagined and contemporary storytelling. We provide a platform for new writing and interdisciplinary work, aiming to give voice to the underrepresented and challenge perceptions. Since opening in 2013 notable in-house productions include *Woyzeck* (2013), *Macbeth* (2014), *Colour* (2015) *Mule* (2016), *Spring Offensive* (2017) and *Zeraffa Giraffa* (2017). Omnibus Theatre is led by Artistic Director Marie McCarthy. Patrons include Dame Judi Dench, Sir Michael Gambon, Matthew Warchus, Sir Richard Eyre and Maggi Hambling. We are a registered charity and receive no core funding.

Omnibus_theatre | @Omnibus_Theatre

Hearing Things was first performed at the Albany Theatre, Deptford on Tuesday 26th of April 2016.

NICHOLAS	David Annen
JANET/GRACE/HOPE	Jeanette Rourke
INOCENT/PATRICK	Seun Shote

Director	Jim Pope
Designers	Miriam Nabarro
	and Jemima Robinson
Sound designer	Becky Smith
Stage Manager/DSM	Holly Marsh
Dramaturg	Lin Coghlan
Producer	Nadezhda Zhelyazkova

And subsequently at Omnibus Theatre, Clapham on Tuesday 31st January 2017

NICHOLAS	Jim Pope
JANET/GRACE/HOPE	Jeanette Rourke
INNOCENT/PATRICK	Daniel Ward

Director	Jim Pope
Assistant Director	Robert Hale
Stage Manager/	
Production Manager	Gareth Howells

The writer would like to thank staff and clients at Music and Change, staff and patients at Homerton University Hospital and at The Maudsley Hospital, Michael Amaning, Jeanette Rourke, Segun Olaiya, Suzanna Whitefield, Marvin Blair, Dreamer, Mike Alfreds, Nina Ward and the Royal Literary fund for financial support.

Thanks also to Lin Coghlan for sound and inspiring dramaturgy and to Jim Pope, without whose determination, hard work and vision the play would not have been written.

INNOCENT, with his mother HOPE, and NICHOLAS, with his father PATRICK, are there as children. So for NICHOLAS it is 1980, and for INNOCENT it is 2006.

INNOCENT is eating some watermelon. He has a towel and a football.

HOPE: Why don't you go and play with that boy over there?

    INNOCENT looks at NICHOLAS.

    Innocent.

    He looks at her.

    Go on. Ask him if he wants some watermelon.

    INNOCENT shakes his head.

    He's building a sandcastle.

    INNOCENT looks.

    You want to build a sandcastle?

    INNOCENT shakes his head.

    How are you ever going to make friends in this country if you won't talk to anyone. Mmmm?

    He doesn't respond. Sound of young children laughing.

    Your sister has made a little friend.

    INNOCENT looks at his four-year-old sister and her friend.

    You have to make an effort Innocent.

    INNOCENT puts his towel over his head. HOPE lies back in the sand.

    NICHOLAS has buried his father in the sand. He flicks sand at him.

PATRICK: Careful lad.

1

NICHOLAS giggles and flicks more sand.

Nicholas! I told you. Careful!

NICHOLAS stops. He climbs on top of PATRICK.

Uff. You're heavy.

NICHOLAS: You're a big old sandman.

PATRICK: Am I?

NICHOLAS: A big old smelly sandman. And you got fat from eating too much chips and ice-cream.

PATRICK: That sounds like a little boy that I know.

NICHOLAS: And doughnuts and coke and you just don't know when you've had enough. That's why you're so fat.

PATRICK: Is that true?

NICHOLAS: And you got so fat you had to lie down in the sand to sleep.

PATRICK: Did I?

NICHOLAS: And when you were sleeping a seagle came—

PATRICK: Sea-gull. It's seagull.

NICHOLAS: A seagle came and pecked out your eyes.

INNOCENT is watching.

NICHOLAS gets sand in PATRICK's eyes.

PATRICK: Nicholas! Aowh. That was naughty.

NICHOLAS is stopped in his tracks.

I told you to be careful.

He sits up. NICHOLAS is distressed that the sand is coming off him.

NICHOLAS: No!

He tries to cover him again with sand.

PATRICK: Stop it, Nicholas. That's enough. You've got sand in my eyes.

NICHOLAS stops.

You always have to take things too far. Don't you?

NICHOLAS doesn't respond.

Daddy's going to have to go and wash all this sand off. You want to come?

NICHOLAS doesn't respond.

Come on, I'll buy you an ice cream.

NICHOLAS doesn't respond.

Come on.

NICHOLAS looks at the floor.

Don't you want an ice-cream?

NICHOLAS shrugs.

Don't be a little baby.

NICHOLAS frowns.

Well if you can't be bothered to talk to me then I can't be bothered to talk to you.

He goes.

NICHOLAS flicks sand with his spade.

INNOCENT watches him.

NICHOLAS continues to flick sand. Some of it goes near INNOCENT.

They look at each other.

NICHOLAS flicks more sand.

INNOCENT flicks sand back.

NICHOLAS flicks sand.

INNOCENT flicks sand.

NICHOLAS giggles.

They continue flicking sand.

INNOCENT giggles.

They stop.

INNOCENT holds out a slice of watermelon.

NICHOLAS looks at him.

INNOCENT holds it out.

NICHOLAS takes it.

They both eat sitting a few feet away from each other.

Seagulls.

NICHOLAS: How are you today?

JANET: I'm ok. Fuck off.

NICHOLAS: Pardon?

JANET: Been at the old scratchy, scratchy. The old flights of fancy. The streams of fucking consciousness.

NICHOLAS: You've been writing?

JANET: Yes. Fuck off.

NICHOLAS: Good. How's that going?

JANET: Good, yeah. Fuck off.

NICHOLAS: You seem calmer today.

JANET laughs.

NICHOLAS: What's funny?

JANET: Saw the monkey on your shoulder.

NICHOLAS: You can see a monkey on my shoulder?

JANET laughs.

NICHOLAS: What's going on?

JANET: I don't know. What's going on?

NICHOLAS: You said there was a monkey on my shoulder.

JANET: What you think this is? A fucking circus? A fucking sideshow? A fucking fairground attraction? Roll up, roll up, come and see the fucking monkey crapping on the man's shoulder? Fucking bonkers. He's got monkey shit all down his back. That monkey's an evil bastard, he's got leery eyes. He leers at you that monkey.

NICHOLAS: Yes?

JANET: Fuck off. You should get rid of that monkey.
    He's messing you up good.

NICHOLAS: Is he?

JANET: You strike me as being ok, you know?

NICHOLAS: Thank you.

JANET: You're welcome. Fuck off. But that monkey's got
    his evil eye on you. So everything you do turns to shit.
    Monkey shit all down your back. People can smell it on
    you. You try to be all sort of nice and clean and all sort
    of how are you today but all the time you can see the
    monkey shit steaming off you. You think you can hide it
    but you can't.

NICHOLAS: But is there really a monkey on my back?

    JANET laughs.

    What's funny?

JANET: You are.

NICHOLAS: Am I?

JANET: Are you?

NICHOLAS: I'm asking you.

JANET: I'm asking you.

NICHOLAS: Is it because there's a monkey on my shoulder?

JANET: How long have you been seeing a monkey on your
    shoulder?

NICHOLAS: It's what you said.

JANET: It's what you said.

NICHOLAS: Because you said it first.

JANET: You thought I meant a real one?

NICHOLAS: It was a metaphorical monkey?

JANET: If you say so.

NICHOLAS: So it wasn't real, this monkey?

JANET: No. That would be mad.

(Impersonating a monkey.)

Oooh ooh, ahh, ahh ahh.

He laughs.

Tell me something. You're an educated man, right?

NICHOLAS: You could say so.

JANET: Would you say so?

NICHOLAS: Yes. I went to University.

JANET: So you've got letters after your name?

NICHOLAS: Some.

JANET: BA.

NICHOLAS: Yes.

JANET: MA.

NICHOLAS: MBBch.

JANET: OBE.

NICHOLAS: No.

JANET: BS. FA. LMAO.

NICHOLAS smiles.

7

I always wanted letters after my name. The only ones I got was CAT B.

NICHOLAS: When you were in Holloway.

JANET: My University.

NICHOLAS: Mmmm.

JANET: Not quite Oxbridge. What I don't understand is why you've ended up in here.

NICHOLAS: It's a fair question. But we're not here to talk about me.

JANET: You must admit it's not exactly the best of places to spend your days. I thought my cleaning job was bad enough. But what you do! Couldn't you get anything better? I mean when you were a kid, did you think oh yeah when I grow up I want to go and spend my days in locked wards in falling down hospitals that no fucker wants to spend any money on because there isn't any money to be made from locking up mad people. So every day you have to sit in this shit-hole listening to people like me.

NICHOLAS: What are people like you?

JANET: Fuck off.

GRACE is working on next Sunday's sermon. She has a Bible. NICHOLAS is drinking wine.

NICHOLAS: So they want to put her on a depot.

GRACE: Who do?

NICHOLAS: The pharmacist! I told you, Grace.

GRACE: Oh yes.

NICHOLAS: And Jonas.

GRACE: Jonas?

NICHOLAS: The ward manager.

GRACE: Why's it called a depot?

NICHOLAS: What?

GRACE: It's a funny word.

NICHOLAS: The drug gets administered in way that keeps it stored at the site of the injection.

GRACE: Oh depot as in bus depot!

NICHOLAS: Yes. So it can be absorbed over a prolonged period.

GRACE: So why does Jonah–?

NICHOLAS: Jonas.

GRACE: Why does Jonas want to put her on a depot?

NICHOLAS: He keeps banging on about her being non-compliant and saying a depot is the only way of guaranteeing that she takes her meds. The woman's got a phobia of needles for God's sake. But he just wants her drugged and out to free up her bed.

GRACE: That's terrible.

NICHOLAS: Of course it is! But given the number of bed places that have been cut in mental health it's kind of understandable. You've got people being sent from Cornwall to Cumbria because there are no beds in the local area.

GRACE: *(Engrossed in her writing.)* Mmmm.

NICHOLAS: They get arrested by the police and there are no beds to put them in. The police don't want a psychotic person in their cells. So they get sent to prison.

GRACE: Would you have diagnosed Abraham as a schizophrenic?

NICHOLAS: What!?

GRACE: You know, God told him to sacrifice his son but at the last moment he provided a ram caught in a thicket–

NICHOLAS: I do know the story of Abraham and Isaac.

GRACE: In religious terms it's accepted that God reveals himself and talks to us.

NICHOLAS: Why are we talking about this?

GRACE: My sermon this week is about how God tests us.

NICHOLAS rolls his eyes. He pours himself more wine.

GRACE pauses to look at how much he is drinking.

NICHOLAS: It's all about numbers. The government imposes these bloody targets on us but they don't fucking ring-fence the funding to make the improvements in the service.

GRACE's mobile rings. She looks at it.

Who is it?

GRACE: Dorothy Grainger.

NICHOLAS groans.

I ought to take it.

NICHOLAS: Grace!

GRACE: What?

NICHOLAS: Do you have to talk to her now?

GRACE: She's bereaved.

NICHOLAS: It's the one evening you've been home this week.

GRACE: OK.

She dismisses the call and returns to her sermon.

NICHOLAS: Talking therapy is really helping her.

GRACE: Janet?

NICHOLAS: Yes. Medication has its place but there are advantages to her not being practically comatose. And she'll probably be discharged just as quickly through the work I'm doing with her. Talking therapies don't get a look in. Too labour intensive. Too expensive. And the fucking IAPT is so outcome- and data-driven.

GRACE: IAPT?

NICHOLAS: I told you that.

GRACE: I don't remember.

NICHOLAS: Hundreds of times.

GRACE: Sorry.

NICHOLAS: Improving Access to Psychological Therapies.

GRACE: Right.

She continues with her notes.

NICHOLAS: It all comes down to the fucking market.

Every time he swears GRACE winces slightly.

Invent a better anti-depressant and you can sell it to prescribers and make a profit. How do you market talking therapy? The IAPT outcomes are all about returning patients to their place in society so that they become productive – whatever that means. They don't give points for helping the patient work out what they want from their fucking life.

GRACE: I hate it when you get drunk and start swearing.

NICHOLAS: Oh fuck off.

She says nothing. He feels abashed.

Sorry Vicar.

They look at each other.

GRACE's mobile rings.

GRACE: It's her again.

NICHOLAS: Go on take it.

She leaves the room with the mobile.

He pours himself more wine.

NICHOLAS AND PATRICK 1

PATRICK is sitting in a deck chair. Seagulls.

PATRICK: More wine?

NICHOLAS: No thanks.

PATRICK: Please yourself.

He pours himself a glass.

So to what do we owe this unexpected and rare visit?

NICHOLAS: No reason.

PATRICK: Don't tell me you've suddenly developed a concern for your father.

NICHOLAS: I would never do that.

PATRICK: Hah! Your mother been talking, has she?

NICHOLAS: What?

PATRICK: Your mother ask you to come?

NICHOLAS doesn't answer.

PATRICK: Thought so.

NICHOLAS: She's worried about you. Says you've been forgetting things.

PATRICK: For God's sake. The trouble with you lot is you read too much into things.

NICHOLAS: What happened last week? She said you couldn't find your way home.

PATRICK: I was on my way back from my conference in Cambridge and I got lost.

NICHOLAS: Dad! She said it took you eight hours.

PATRICK: Every exit on the M25 looks the same.

NICHOLAS: What were you doing on the M25?

PATRICK: Very interesting conference. About the latest developments in gene therapy for the treatment of cancer.

NICHOLAS: You're keeping your hand in then?

PATRICK: I saw your friend from Uni there.

NICHOLAS: Graham.

PATRICK: Hmmm?

NICHOLAS: Graham Lloyd.

PATRICK: Oh yes. It's really cutting edge stuff. And he's at the forefront of it.

NICHOLAS: Lot of money and resources in Cancer Research.

PATRICK: Don't start. Vanessa not with you?

NICHOLAS: Who?

PATRICK: Your um... she's your wife.

NICHOLAS: Grace.

PATRICK: Grace yes. I meant Grace.

NICHOLAS: Vanessa was years ago. At Oxford.

PATRICK: So how are things at the asylum?

NICHOLAS: Fine.

PATRICK: Is that all I'm getting?

NICHOLAS: What more do you want?

PATRICK: A few tales of madness and delusion to relieve the boredom. I look forward to the latest episodes. Better than a soap.

NICHOLAS: I aim to please.

PATRICK: Can't say I've ever noticed.

NICHOLAS: Ha ha.

PATRICK: Trouble with being retired is one's stock of stories about one's patients and their extraordinary antics doesn't get renewed.

NICHOLAS: Nothing to talk to your golfing buddies about on the walk to the green?

PATRICK: Ha. Your friend Graham plays you know. Invited me to a game when I'm next in Cambridge.

NICHOLAS: Great.

PATRICK: Marvellous bloke. He's involved in this research about gene therapy.

NICHOLAS: You said.

PATRICK: Come on! What's the point of coming to see me if you don't entertain me?

NICHOLAS: I see my patients as more than sources of anecdotes for the golf course.

PATRICK: That's my wrist firmly slapped.

NICHOLAS: Sorry.

PATRICK: You need to lighten up.

NICHOLAS: I do.

PATRICK: If you work in the "caring professions" you have to give yourself a break sometimes.

NICHOLAS: A break from caring?

PATRICK: Makes you a better physician. Having a sense of humour. It's needed. Especially in your line of work.

NICHOLAS: Yes it's a laugh a minute.

PATRICK: Even oncology wasn't all doom and gloom.

NICHOLAS: I'm sure you managed to find the funny side of tumours.

PATRICK: Your friend Graham. Great sense of humour. Just been to Africa. Had to work in appalling conditions. Had me in stitches. Didn't stop him getting the job done. He's looking into eliminating the Hepatits B virus out there to prevent the emergence of liver cancer.

NICHOLAS: I can see his knighthood coming any time now.

PATRICK: There are a lot of people alive today in Mali thanks to his attentions.

NICHOLAS: He can afford to slum it once in a while.

PATRICK: Eh?

NICHOLAS: The packet he makes from private practice.

PATRICK: Nothing shameful about making money.

NICHOLAS: How's Mum?

PATRICK: Didn't you see her up at the house?

NICHOLAS: Yes.

PATRICK: The thing that gets me about people who bellyache about the privatization of the NHS is they can't admit that market forces improve efficiency and productivity.

NICHOLAS: I thought she was looking tired.

PATRICK: Who?

NICHOLAS: Mum.

PATRICK: It's a different world to 1948. There are more of us oldies for one thing. We can't go on hemorrhaging money.

NICHOLAS: You really want a two-tier health system?

PATRICK: People have to stop expecting to get it all for nothing as a bloody right.

NICHOLAS: Well I can tell you one thing: the money isn't hemorrhaging very fast into mental health.

PATRICK: Here we go! Soapbox time.

NICHOLAS: Dad, do you know what percentage of NHS funding mental health gets?

PATRICK: I'm sure you're going to tell me.

NICHOLAS: Ten per cent.

PATRICK: Sounds quite a bit to me.

NICHOLAS: Except that mental health accounts for twenty-eight per cent of the illness burden.

PATRICK: Well we know why that is.

NICHOLAS: Do we?

PATRICK: Too many silly buggers telling people they're depressed when they're having a bad day.

NICHOLAS: Ah. Is that what it is?

Pause. Seagulls.

PATRICK: Hmmm. Love this time of day.

NICHOLAS: It's nice. Always liked it here.

PATRICK: You should bring Vanessa next time.

NICHOLAS: Yes?

PATRICK: Lovely girl.

NICHOLAS: Yes.

NICHOLAS: So what was the trigger?

JANET: Jonas telling me I had to go on a depot.

NICHOLAS: And what did that make you feel?

JANET: What do you think it made me feel? Fucking angry.

NICHOLAS: Right. What else?

JANET: Fear.

NICHOLAS: Yes.

JANET: Murderous.

NICHOLAS: OK. That all?

JANET: It's enough isn't it?

NICHOLAS: So what thoughts did you have?

JANET: I want to kill the fucker.

NICHOLAS: *(Looking at her.)* Uh huh.

JANET: What?

NICHOLAS: Any other thoughts?

JANET: I know what you want me to say.

NICHOLAS: Do you?

JANET: Stop doing that!

NICHOLAS: Doing what?

JANET: That!

NICHOLAS: Tell me what I'm doing.

JANET: Throwing things back at me by asking questions.

19

NICHOLAS: Is that what I'm–?

He stops himself. They laugh.

What do you think I want you to say?

JANET: That it made me want to top myself.

NICHOLAS: You're mindreading. I don't want you to say that. Not unless it's true.

JANET: Right.

NICHOLAS: Is it true?

JANET: Would be fucking stupid to admit it wouldn't it?

NICHOLAS: Not if it's true. I need to get an accurate picture of how you are at the moment.

JANET: Alright!! Yes I did have that thought. But that doesn't mean I'd do it.

NICHOLAS: Of course. Any other thoughts.

JANET: Nicholas has stitched me up.

NICHOLAS: OK. Any others?

She shakes her head.

So what did you make it mean?

She looks at him.

NICHOLAS: Mmmm?

JANET: That every fucker is against me.

NICHOLAS: OK.

JANET: That I can't trust anyone. That nobody's ever going to see me as anything but a fucking loony.

NICHOLAS: Right.

JANET: That I'm never going to be well again. That I'm useless. That everything in my life is shit.

He nods.

NICHOLAS: So let's look at those. Is everyone really against you?

JANET: It feels like it.

NICHOLAS: But are they? Really? Am I against you?

JANET: I don't know.

NICHOLAS: OK so you don't know. So actually everyone might not be against you.

JANET: I suppose.

NICHOLAS: So what are you doing?

JANET: Catastrophising.

NICHOLAS: Good.

JANET: Tick.

NICHOLAS: What else was it? That you're never going to be well again. Do you know that for a fact?

JANET: I don't know that I will get better.

NICHOLAS: But in the past you've been ill and you've recovered.

JANET: OK.

NICHOLAS: So?

JANET: Fortune-telling.

NICHOLAS: Yes.

JANET: Two ticks.

NICHOLAS: Are you useless? Is everything in your life shit?

JANET: Go on tell me why not.

NICHOLAS: Why is Donna with you?

JANET: Eh?

NICHOLAS: Donna. She visits you every day. She obviously cares a lot about you. Why does she do that?

JANET: She feels sorry for me.

NICHOLAS: She doesn't have to stick by you. What does she get out of it?

JANET: I'm a good fuck.

NICHOLAS: Right. So you're not useless. As a sexual partner you have your uses.

JANET: Ha.

NICHOLAS: But I suspect that you have other qualities that make her want to be with you.

JANET: Like my bullshit detector.

NICHOLAS: Like your perceptiveness and your intelligence.

JANET: OK. OK. I was catastrophising again.

NICHOLAS: But can you see that these are all mental habits?

JANET: So all I need to do is have a more positive attitude and all my problems will disappear. I just need to buck myself up and then I'll stop being a burden on everyone. They'll be able to send me back to work and everything will be fucking hunky-dory.

NICHOLAS: You know that's not what I think. I want you to regain some control over your life.

JANET: Being forced to take my meds with a needle won't give me much control.

NICHOLAS: No it won't.

She looks at him.

Why do you think I've stitched you up?

JANET: Because I'm perceptive and intelligent!

NICHOLAS: Meaning?

JANET: You must have given the nod for me to go on a depot.

NICHOLAS: You're mindreading again.

JANET: Yes I fucking am.

NICHOLAS: Except that I've recommended that you stay on oral medication with a view to being discharged.

JANET: Oh.

NICHOLAS: I want you to start managing your medication yourself. Start recognizing when you are getting ill and need help.

JANET: Jonas must have been pretty pissed off.

NICHOLAS: I persuaded everyone on the Ward Round that it was for the best.

She nods.

So tell me about those feelings.

JANET: What about them?

NICHOLAS: Have any of them changed?

JANET: Well I don't want to murder you any more.

NICHOLAS: Tick.

They laugh.

23

HOPE: It began when he got into his late teenage years. When
he was a boy he was quiet – not noisy like his friends,
not a loudmouth. He generally kept himself to himself.
He was shy. And then as he got older he spent more
and more time in his room. They all do that, don't they?
Talking to each other on their Playstations. But then he
started refusing to go out. He must have been fifteen.
There was a lot of gang activity on the estate at that time.
Drug dealers. And then that boy was killed, stabbed. So to
be honest with you, I was relieved that he wanted to stay
at home with me and his sister.

NICHOLAS: You say there were drugs on the estate?

HOPE: Yes.

NICHOLAS: Did Innocent take drugs?

HOPE: We always told him about the dangers.

NICHOLAS: We?

HOPE: Pardon?

NICHOLAS: You mean you and Innocent's father?

HOPE: My husband has businesses in Ghana. So he was
unable to be with us for much of the time.

NICHOLAS: I see.

HOPE: Import/export, you know? And we still have family
over there. Boys need a man's guidance, don't you think?

NICHOLAS: I do.

HOPE: So I thought, if he is in his room, he isn't running the
streets getting into trouble. He is safe.

NICHOLAS: Yes.

HOPE: When we first arrived in London, things were hard. I am a nurse and the only work I could get was with an agency. I had to work shifts and so I was not always there after school. Innocent was about thirteen and his sister was seven. Sometimes he had to pick her up from school and give her tea. He was very good with her. He had to grow up very quickly. He never complained.

She wipes her eyes.

NICHOLAS: I'm sure you did your very best.

HOPE: Then I got a job in a home for the elderly and I had more control over my hours. I was able to be there for them. But maybe the damage was already done.

NICHOLAS: To be honest with you Mrs Asamoah–

HOPE: Please, call me Hope.

NICHOLAS: To be honest with you Hope, we don't know what causes these psychotic incidents. We know that there can be triggers but these are often about chemical imbalances and are not necessarily related to psychological trauma.

HOPE: That first time, he was not sleeping and he wouldn't let me into his room. He had covered the walls and the window with silver paper, you know the metal foil that you use in the oven. He said it was to stop the rays from the mobile phone masts and I had heard that some people are very sensitive to the rays from them. Have you heard that?

NICHOLAS: Yes – it's microwave radiation but I don't think–

HOPE: But then he started to talk about the voices that were coming to him and they were telling him things about his father and Osama Bin Laden. Crazy things, you know?

NICHOLAS: Yes. I read that in the notes.

HOPE: It was very upsetting. He started saying terrible
things about his father. That he was responsible for what
happened in New York when the aeroplanes crashed into
the World Trade Center. Really crazy. But I still didn't
understand what was going on. I tried to reason with him
but he wouldn't listen. I didn't realize he was sick. It is
very frightening when someone starts to say these things.
You think maybe you are becoming crazy yourself.
I thought I was going crazy.

NICHOLAS: That's very common.

HOPE: None of us were getting any sleep. It was terrible.

NICHOLAS: It must have been.

HOPE: He was convinced that the FBI was watching him and
that they were going to take his sister away. He phoned
me at work one day and told me that I had to come home
because there were people outside the flat and they were
trying to get in and they were going to take Precious and
we would never see her again. When I arrived home the
house was empty. It was the worst time. Then the police
phoned. Innocent and Precious were on the railway
bridge over the canal and he was threatening to jump.
I knew then that we needed help. I couldn't let him put
my daughter's life in danger. I had no choice.

NICHOLAS: Indeed you didn't.

HOPE: It was the hardest thing. To hand my son over like
that and ask that he be kept a prisoner in a locked facility.
I could never have imagined that I would have to do such
a thing.

NICHOLAS: It's very hard.

She weeps.

NICHOLAS: So would you try that?

INNOCENT doesn't respond.

Innocent?

INNOCENT looks at him.

Would you try that?

INNOCENT: OK.

NICHOLAS: If you hear a voice just put your hand up and I'll tell it to stop talking to you.

INNOCENT doesn't respond.

OK?

INNOCENT: Yes.

He hears a voice and responds but doesn't put his hand up.

NICHOLAS: What's going on?

No response.

Are you hearing something now?

INNOCENT: I want to see my sister.

NICHOLAS: Is it your sister you can hear?

INNOCENT: No.

NICHOLAS: So what is the voice saying?

INNOCENT: I can't tell you.

NICHOLAS: OK. Why can't you tell me?

INNOCENT: They'll take her away.

NICHOLAS: Do you believe the voice, Innocent?

INNOCENT: I don't know.

NICHOLAS: So the next time you hear the voice put your hand up.

INNOCENT nods.

He puts his hand up.

Stop it. Stop it.

His hand is still up.

Can you still hear the voice?

INNOCENT: No.

NICHOLAS: So if the voice stops, bring your hand down, like you did last time.

INNOCENT brings his hand down.

And if the voice comes back just raise your arm again and I'll–

INNOCENT raises his arm.

Stop it. Stop it.

INNOCENT's arm starts to come down.

Right.

INNOCENT raises his arm again.

Stop it. Stop it. Stop it.

His hand slowly comes down.

OK?

INNOCENT: Yes.

NICHOLAS: Right, so the next time you hear the voice I want you to shout "stop it" until it goes away. You're going to shout. You remember this from last time?

INNOCENT: Yes.

He puts his hand up.

NICHOLAS: Tell it to stop.

INNOCENT: *(Quietly.)* Stop it.

NICHOLAS: Nice and loud.

INNOCENT: Stop it! Stop it!

NICHOLAS: Good.

INNOCENT: Stop it! Stop it! Stop it!

His hand slowly comes down.

NICHOLAS: Right. Very good. You don't have to raise your arm any more. That was just so I knew you were hearing the voice.

INNOCENT shoots his arm up.

INNOCENT: Stop it! Stop it! Stop it!

He brings his hand down.

Pause.

NICHOLAS: Good. You're doing really well. This time if you hear the voice, I want you to whisper "Stop it", instead of shouting.

INNOCENT doesn't respond.

What's happening?

INNOCENT: They're saying they will never let me see her again.

He raises his arm.

NICHOLAS: Just whisper, "Stop it."

INNOCENT: *(Whispering.)* Stop it. Stop it.

He starts to bring his arm down but then raises it again.

NICHOLAS: You don't need to raise your arm.

INNOCENT lowers his arm.

INNOCENT: *(Whispering.)* Stop it. Stop it.

NICHOLAS: Good.

INNOCENT: Stop it. Stop it. Stop it.

Pause.

NICHOLAS: Now the last stage, which we didn't do last time, is just to think, "Stop it!" but not to actually say it out loud at all.

He watches to see if INNOCENT has understood. INNOCENT is unresponsive.

Can you do that?

INNOCENT: Yes.

INNOCENT raises his arm.

NICHOLAS: Don't worry about raising your arm.

INNOCENT is thinking "stop it". NICHOLAS watches him.

How's that.

INNOCENT: They've gone.

NICHOLAS: Great.

INNOCENT: So can I see my sister?

NICHOLAS: We'll talk to your Mum about letting her come
and visit.

INNOCENT: When?

NICHOLAS: Soon.

INNOCENT thinks about this.

INNOCENT: *(Putting his hand up and whispering.)* Stop it.
Stop it. Stop it.

JANET: You come for the writing group?

INNOCENT: Writing group?

JANET: There's this OT, Sam, he runs a writing group in here on Thursdays.

INNOCENT: Oh I see.

There is a noise outside the room on the ward.

JANET: Mad here, isn't it?

INNOCENT: Yes.

JANET: And that's just the staff.

INNOCENT: Pardon?

JANET: Who's your shrink?

INNOCENT: My…?

JANET: Psychiatrist. Hate the fuckers.

INNOCENT: Oh yes. Dr Hamilton.

JANET: Oh Nicholas. Watch him. He likes to pretend he's on our side.

INNOCENT puts his hand up and thinks "Stop it!"

You ok?

He brings his arm down again.

INNOCENT: Yes, I'm fine.

He puts his arm up again. She watches.

He brings his arm down.

JANET: The old "stop it" routine didn't do it for me.

INNOCENT: I used to like to write in school.

JANET: You should come along.

INNOCENT: But it got me into trouble.

JANET: How come?

INNOCENT: The things I wrote upset my teachers. They said I was crazy.

JANET: You're in good company.

INNOCENT: I'm sorry?

JANET: Ezra Pound, Sylvia Plath, Virginia Woolf, Ernest Hemingway. Even Leo Tolstoy.

INNOCENT: These people were all crazy?

JANET: Bi-polar, depressive, schizophrenic, suicidal. All or any of the above.

INNOCENT: I saw *War and Peace* on television.

JANET: Tolstoy, famous depressive, nearly topped himself but found God instead. Creative people and schizophrenics have a lower density of dopamine receptors. Their brains don't filter out information and that helps them to make connections no sane person would make.

INNOCENT: Is this true?

JANET: Gospel. What they got you on?

INNOCENT: Olanzapine.

JANET: Snap. Luckily they hadn't discovered it when all those writers were around. They'd have all been overweight diabetics who were too comatose to write a fucking word. Don't tell Nicholas I said that.

INNOCENT: Of course not.

JANET: Sometimes it helps. But sometimes it feels that the side-effects are worse than having the illness.

INNOCENT: Yes! That is so true! That is exactly how I feel.

JANET: Yeah well, best keep it to yourself. They don't like being called drug pushers.

INNOCENT: You are funny.

JANET: Yep. Funny in the head, that's me.

INNOCENT: No I mean you make me laugh,

JANET: Good.

They look at each other.

I'm Janet.

INNOCENT: Hello Janet. I am Innocent.

JANET: What of?

INNOCENT: Oh yes!

JANET: Sorry. You must be sick of that joke.

INNOCENT: Good to meet you Janet.

JANET: So you going to come to this writing group?

INNOCENT: Yes, maybe I will.

NICHOLAS: So what do you think?

JANET: Yes.

NICHOLAS: Every other group – women, black people, gay people, the disabled – they can speak for themselves – they don't need anyone to advocate for them. That's not true for mental health service users.

JANET: I hate the way people make up new ways of saying you're fucking mad. Service users!

NICHOLAS: Mad people as a group aren't allowed to advocate for themselves.

JANET: I don't want to be part of a group.

NICHOLAS: That's understandable given the stigma involved.

JANET: Donna says I'm apolitical.

NICHOLAS: Does she?

JANET: She's always on a soapbox.

NICHOLAS: Why does she say you're apolitical?

JANET: Why do they call it that?

NICHOLAS: Apolitical?

JANET: Why a soapbox?

NICHOLAS: I think it goes back to when people at Speakers' Corner would take a box with them to stand on.

JANET: Why a soapbox though? Why not a tea box or an orange box?

NICHOLAS: Any box that has been used for transporting dry goods.

JANET: Why soap though? I mean you wouldn't think that's the most common commodity.

NICHOLAS: No.

JANET: That there'd be hundreds of them lying around waiting for someone to come and use them to stand on.

NICHOLAS: Look. I understand why you might not want to stand up and represent mental health patients. That's the awful double bind.

JANET: Double bind.

NICHOLAS: It describes a situation where an individual receives two conflicting messages, and one message negates the other, creating a dilemma that she is unable to escape.

JANET: Like when you said that if I didn't accept that I was ill, then you wouldn't be able to say I was well enough to come off section.

NICHOLAS: Did I say that?

JANET: You've not got a very good memory. You'd only let me out if I said I was too ill to be let out.

NICHOLAS: A classic double bind.

JANET: And then when I got angry they said my anger was a sign that I was mad. And I had to be sedated.

NICHOLAS: Yes.

JANET: Anyone would get angry about being kept somewhere against their will.

NICHOLAS: True.

JANET: That's a fucking double bind if there ever was one.

NICHOLAS: Janet, you're very clear about the issues. That's why I think you'd make a great advocate.

JANET: And it would be a feather in your cap, wouldn't it?

NICHOLAS: Maybe.

JANET: No Nicholas. Not doing it. If I stand up shouting my mouth off about patients' rights what's to stop people saying I'm a bloody loony?

NICHOLAS: An advocate doesn't have to shout their mouth off.

JANET: No. Once I'm out of here the last thing I want is to come back in and be a fucking advocate for some other loony.

NICHOLAS: That's because of the stigma.

JANET: Yes. It creates a double bind, doesn't it Nicholas?

NICHOLAS: It does.

JANET: So you still going to let me out?

NICHOLAS: Of course.

GRACE: "I feel emotionally drained by my work."

NICHOLAS: Yes.

GRACE: Once a week?

NICHOLAS: More than that.

GRACE: A few times a week?

NICHOLAS: Every day.

GRACE: Right, 6. "Working with people all day long requires a great deal of effort."

NICHOLAS: It certainly does.

GRACE: Nicholas!

NICHOLAS: What?

GRACE: How often?

NICHOLAS: Not every day but more than once a week.

GRACE: 5. "I feel as if my work is breaking me down."

NICHOLAS: Mmmm. A few times a month.

GRACE: 3.

NICHOLAS: No once a week.

GRACE: 4. "I feel frustrated in my work."

NICHOLAS: So did all these vicars sit round doing this test on your retreat?

GRACE: Not all of us.

NICHOLAS: How did you score?

GRACE: I'm far from burnt out.

NICHOLAS: When you're on the other end of these
    questionnaires you realize how crude they are.

GRACE: "I feel frustrated in my work."

NICHOLAS: Every day.

GRACE: Every day?

NICHOLAS: Yes.

GRACE: Alright. 6. I don't think it's that often.

NICHOLAS: I'm sure you're not meant to question my
    answers.

GRACE: "I feel I work too hard at my job."

NICHOLAS: I don't know about that.

GRACE: You do work too hard.

NICHOLAS: You do. I feel I don't work hard enough.

GRACE: So?

NICHOLAS: Once a month.

GRACE: OK, 2. Section B. Depersonalization. "I feel I look
    after certain parishioners – uh patients – impersonally as if
    they are objects."

NICHOLAS: Every day at the moment.

GRACE: You're very hard on yourself. "I feel tired when I get
    up in the morning and have to face another day at work."

NICHOLAS: Yes every bloody day.

GRACE: "I have the feeling that my parishioners – that
    my patients – make me responsible for some of their
    problems."

NICHOLAS: All their bloody problems.

GRACE: "I am at the end of patience at the end of my working day."

NICHOLAS: Most days.

GRACE: "I really don't care about what happens to some of my… patients."

He doesn't know how to answer.

You do care.

NICHOLAS: Not at the moment.

GRACE: I don't believe that.

He shrugs.

NICHOLAS: You want to answer for me?

GRACE: No.

NICHOLAS: Once a week.

GRACE: "I have become insensitive to people."

NICHOLAS: You think I have.

GRACE: I don't.

NICHOLAS: You said I'm self-obsessed.

GRACE: Perhaps this wasn't a good idea.

NICHOLAS: A few times a week.

GRACE: "I'm afraid that my ministry is making me uncaring."

Pause.

He starts to cry.

Nicholas.

NICHOLAS: I am. I don't have…

GRACE: It's the job. High work demands without adequate resources. Responsibility without authority.

NICHOLAS: Yes, yes. Been there, got the badge.

GRACE: You said yourself, "psychiatrists are prone to internalize stress".

NICHOLAS: Blah blah.

GRACE: I'm not the enemy, Nick.

He doesn't respond.

She looks at her watch.

It's late.

NICHOLAS: Mmmm.

GRACE: You coming up?

He shrugs like the ten-year-old NICHOLAS.

Night then.

She goes to kiss him. He avoids.

NICHOLAS: Night.

PATRICK is in the deckchair as before.

PATRICK: Ahhh!

GRACE: Hello Patrick!

PATRICK: Ah it's um…

GRACE: Grace.

PATRICK: Yes. The lady vicar.

GRACE: Just vicar will do.

PATRICK: Ah yes. No-one says lady doctor any more either. Nicholas with you?

GRACE: No. Just me today. I was on my way back from a meeting in Ely and I thought I'd call in.

PATRICK: Oh yes? You going to be the next bishop?

GRACE: Hardly.

PATRICK: I suppose Nick's at work today anyway.

GRACE: Well…

PATRICK: Haven't seen hide nor hair of him for months.

GRACE: He came up to see you the other week.

PATRICK: Apart from then, I mean. Did he send you to spy on me?

GRACE: Spy on you?

PATRICK: His mother thinks I'm going senile.

Pause.

Trouble with psychiatrists is that they think they know
better than you what's going on in your head.

GRACE: Isn't that true of oncologists too? You tell people
they're ill when they feel well.

PATRICK: Touché! What do vicars know that the rest of us
don't?

GRACE: That only God knows best.

PATRICK: Ha!

GRACE: He's not at work actually. Nick.

PATRICK: No?

GRACE: He's off sick.

PATRICK: What's he got? Man-flu?

GRACE: It's stress.

PATRICK: Stress! Spending Time Relaxing Expecting Salary
Still.

GRACE: Seems there's nothing wrong with your mind.

PATRICK: Stress covers a multitude of sins.

GRACE: He's very overworked.

PATRICK: Everybody's overworked.

GRACE: And under-resourced.

PATRICK: Don't know why he chose psychiatry.

GRACE: He believes he can help people.

PATRICK snorts.

You were a hard act to follow Patrick.

PATRICK: Oh so this is my fault?

GRACE: Of course not.

PATRICK: He always was over-sensitive.

GRACE: That's what makes him a good psychiatrist.

PATRICK: All those years studying medicine just to throw it away on a branch of the profession that has no scientific basis. They make it up as they go along.

GRACE: Maybe. Maybe that's all any of us do.

(After a beat.)

I think he feels he's disappointed you.

PATRICK: No grit. He's– what age is he? Thirty-three, thirty-four, is it?

GRACE: *(Alarmed.)* He's forty-six, Patrick.

PATRICK: Course he is. You'd have thought his balls would have dropped by this time.

She nods.

I tried Grace. I did try. It wasn't always easy. The hours I worked. But I tried to be a good father to him.

GRACE: I'm sure you did.

PATRICK: I sometimes think your God is a bit of a sadist. Watching all our desperate endeavours and bringing it all to nothing in the end.

GRACE: You don't have to make it mean that.

PATRICK: You sound like Nicholas.

She smiles.

It doesn't feel like a matter of choice.

44

Sainsburys self-checkout.

NICHOLAS is buying wine.

AUTOMATED VOICE: Notes are dispensed beneath the scanner.

NICHOLAS picks up his bottle.

AUTOMATED VOICE: Thank you for using Sainsburys self-checkout.

He starts to go. JANET is at another machine.

JANET: Nicholas.

NICHOLAS: Ah Janet.

JANET: You exist in the real world!

NICHOLAS: I do indeed.

AUTOMATED VOICE: Place item in bagging area.

JANET: Alright. Alright.

(Looking at his wine.)

Rioja – very nice. You self-medicating?

NICHOLAS: Something like that.

JANET: It's expensive that one.

NICHOLAS: How are you Janet?

JANET: Yeah I'm…

AUTOMATED VOICE: Unexpected item in bagging area.

JANET: What?

AUTOMATED VOICE: Please remove this item from bagging area.

She removes the item.

JANET: Yeah I'm great.

NICHOLAS: That's very good to hear.

AUTOMATED VOICE: Item removed from bagging area.
Return item to bagging area before continuing.

JANET: I don't believe this.

(Putting the item back.)

Yeah I've been… I've been writing…

NICHOLAS: About?

JANET: Madhouses I have known.

NICHOLAS: Ah!

JANET: Still not back at work. I don't feel up to it really. But it
means I've got time to write. Very therapeutic.

AUTOMATED VOICE: Unexpected item in bagging area.

JANET: Ugh!

NICHOLAS: Are you using your own bag?

JANET: No.

NICHOLAS: That's usually what causes–

AUTOMATED VOICE: Remove this item from bagging area.

They laugh.

JANET: *(Raising her arm and whispering.)* Stop it! Stop it!

NICHOLAS: Yes!

She removes the item. They both look at the checkout till.

AUTOMATED VOICE: Please wait for assistance.

They look for the assistant.

NICHOLAS: Well I'd better be–

JANET: Yes.

NICHOLAS: Nice bumping into you.

He starts to go.

JANET: Thank you Nicholas.

NICHOLAS: Pardon?

JANET: I just wanted to– I know I wasn't always the easiest patient.

NICHOLAS: Oh.

JANET: Yeah. I was a fucking pain.

NICHOLAS: I'm glad you're doing ok.

JANET: You really helped.

He looks stricken.

NICHOLAS: I'll see you Janet.

JANET: Yeah.

AUTOMATED VOICE: Have you scanned your Nectar card?

JANET: *(In despair.)* Ugh.

(Trying to get an assistant's attention.)

Scuse me!

NICHOLAS: I'll see you.

JANET: Yeah bye.

He goes.

NICHOLAS is 20 – 1990.

PATRICK: Your mother sent down your swimming things.

NICHOLAS: I don't want to go swimming.

PATRICK: It would do you good.

NICHOLAS: Too cold.

PATRICK: Bracing.

NICHOLAS: Yes.

PATRICK: You're looking better.

   NICHOLAS doesn't say anything.

   Bloody stupid you know. Could have ruined your liver.

NICHOLAS: I know Dad. I'm studying medicine.

PATRICK: I shudder to think what would have happened if Vanessa hadn't found you.

   NICHOLAS doesn't respond.

   We all get low.

NICHOLAS: I don't want to talk about it, Dad.

PATRICK: She was distraught, Vanessa. You want to think about how your actions affect other people. What would it have done to Vanessa and your mother if you'd–

NICHOLAS: I said I don't want to talk about it.

PATRICK: You need to face up to it lad. Face up to the consequences of your actions.

NICHOLAS: You mean like you always do?

PATRICK: Yes. Precisely.

NICHOLAS shakes his head.

Was it a cry for help? Is that what it was? That's what the doctor said.

No response.

I spoke to your moral tutor – Dr Mason. They're keeping your place open for you. He said there's no reason why you shouldn't get a first.

NICHOLAS: I don't know if I want to go back.

PATRICK: What are you? A quitter? That what your are?

NICHOLAS: Yes probably.

PATRICK: Oh for God's sake!

NICHOLAS: What would you have felt?

PATRICK: What?

NICHOLAS: You said how upset Mum and Vanessa would have been.

PATRICK: Is this what this was all about? Punishing me?

NICHOLAS: Yeah.

PATRICK: I'd have been devastated.

NICHOLAS: Relieved more like.

PATRICK: Don't be bloody stupid. What a bloody stupid thing to say.

NICHOLAS: You could have got a divorce, married your nurse, started a new family with her.

PATRICK: I'm not listening to this kind of talk.

NICHOLAS: Now who's not facing up to things?

PATRICK: Look, you little shit, don't blame me for your lack of backbone. This was nothing to do with me.

NICHOLAS: No, you've been a perfect Dad.

PATRICK: Just pull yourself together.

NICHOLAS: Great bedside manner. What do you call patients like me? TBPs?

PATRICK: Total bloody pain just about sums it up.

NICHOLAS: Yep.

They both sit there and fume.

INNOCENT: They called you a healer but in our home we knew you for what you really are. We were your subjects and you were our king. A cruel king who was always changing the rules and always ready to punish us for some new law that we had broken. You were a man of God, a pastor for your flock. For them you were a healer. But not for your wife and not for us your kids. When you laid your hands on us it wasn't healing that was in your mind. And on that night, that fatal night, you shot me in the heart. Then you shot me in the heart. Then you came up close and shot me in the shoulder. Point blank. And I want to ask you, did you hate me so much at that moment? A father gives life. He is not meant to take it away again. Did you hate that I wanted to stop you beating up on Mum? Hate that your son had to protect her from you? So you shot me in the heart and you shot me in the heart then you came up close and shot me in the shoulder. But it was the first shot that was the fatal one. They say you had a tumour that was pressing on your brain. They say that's the reason you lost control. They say you weren't yourself. But I remember the kid hiding in his bed while downstairs the storm was brewing – I remember listening for your step outside my door and I pulled the covers over my head. And when I slept I remember the warmth of my piss as it spread out beneath me. But I would wake to the cold and the wet and a whipping from you. It was no tumour that made you shoot me in the heart and shoot me in the heart then come up close and shoot me in the shoulder. That was you who did that. And there was no healing to save me from your rage.

NICHOLAS: Well! You wrote that?

INNOCENT: Yes. I have been busy while you have been away.

NICHOLAS: So I hear. Sam told me you've been attending the writing class.

INNOCENT: We had to make up a character and I wrote that.

NICHOLAS: It's amazing.

INNOCENT: And it's true. My father used to shout at my mother.

NICHOLAS: Oh, so the person speaking is you?

INNOCENT: Oh no, sorry. It's Marvin.

NICHOLAS: Marvin?

INNOCENT: Marvin Gaye.

NICHOLAS: Oh the king of soul.

INNOCENT: Yes.

NICHOLAS: I heard it through the grapevine.

INNOCENT: Yes. I always liked him.

NICHOLAS: Do you feel an affinity for him?

INNOCENT doesn't respond.

Did your Dad do some of the same things that Marvin's Dad did?

INNOCENT: Yes.

NICHOLAS: So Marvin Gaye used to wet the bed.

INNOCENT: Yes.

NICHOLAS: And his Dad punished him for it.

INNOCENT: Sometimes. One time he got his belt out and and the metal bit cut my skin. I've still got the scar.

NICHOLAS: But this is Marvin, not you.

INNOCENT: Oh yes. Sorry.

NICHOLAS: You don't have to apologise. So some of the same things that happened to Marvin Gaye happened to you.

INNOCENT: Yes.

NICHOLAS: So you used your own experience when you were writing the character?

INNOCENT: Yes. But what happened to me was different.

NICHOLAS: Well your Dad didn't shoot you for a start.

INNOCENT: No. He got the FBI involved to watch me. Because I knew he planned 9/11 and they were trying to cover it up.

NICHOLAS: You think your Dad planned the bombing of the twin towers.

INNOCENT: Yes. The twin towers. Yes.

NICHOLAS: This is something we talked about before I was off, isn't it?

INNOCENT: Yes.

NICHOLAS: What did I say when you talked like that?

INNOCENT: That I am delusional.

NICHOLAS: Why do I say that?

INNOCENT avoids.

Why did I say that it is delusional to believe that your father planned the bombing of the twin towers.

INNOCENT: Because it is not true.

NICHOLAS: Do you agree that it's not true?

INNOCENT: Yes. But then I start to get worried.

NICHOLAS: Why?

INNOCENT: Because the FBI are tracking me with bugs and antennae. They have recording devices that they put in the electrical wires. And they recruit people who pretend to be normal but really they are working for the FBI. There is one of the nurses here. He is an agent.

NICHOLAS: And is that really happening?

INNOCENT: I don't know. It might be.

NICHOLAS: Does Marvin believe that his Dad is working for the FBI?

INNOCENT: No Marvin is not crazy.

NICHOLAS: I see. So when you're being Marvin Gaye you don't have those delusions?

INNOCENT: No.

NICHOLAS: That's interesting.

INNOCENT: What is interesting?

NICHOLAS: That when you're pretending to be Marvin you're not delusional.

INNOCENT: Sam said you had to be somebody else. So even though I think the FBI are watching me I don't bring that into the character.

NICHOLAS: Right. So it sounds as if you know the difference between being ill and being well.

INNOCENT: But the FBI might be there. Maybe Marvin Gaye's father worked for the FBI and he didn't know.

NICHOLAS: But you said that Marvin isn't ill. Which is why he doesn't think his father is an FBI agent. And when you're well, you don't think the FBI is watching you either, do you?

INNOCENT: No. I don't.

Sound of tube station.

JANET stands on the edge of the platform.

STATION ANNOUNCEMENT: This is a safety announcement. Due to today's inclement weather please take extra care whilst on the station. Surfaces may be slippery.

Sound of tube approaching.

STATION ANNOUNCEMENT: Ladies and gentlemen, please stand behind the yellow line on the platform at all times for your safety.

Sound of approaching tube gets louder.

INNOCENT: A happy memory?

NICHOLAS: Yes.

INNOCENT: It was just after we arrived in England. We went to stay with my uncle in Norfolk. He lived by the sea. Every day we went to the beach.

NICHOLAS: You and your mother?

INNOCENT: And my sister. She was about four years old. I was ten.

NICHOLAS: It's lovely the Norfolk coast.

INNOCENT: At first everything was strange. People stared.

NICHOLAS: Because you were different?

INNOCENT: Because we were African.

NICHOLAS: But it was a happy memory.

INNOCENT: I made friends on the beach. There was one boy–

He stops. He holds up a finger.

He takes out his phone.

I am sorry. I cannot speak now. I will phone you later.

He listens.

No. Not now. I will talk to you tonight. At ten 'o' clock. Goodbye.

He put his phone back in his pocket.

NICHOLAS: Very good.

INNOCENT: Yes. If I talk to them like this, they wait.

NICHOLAS: I'm glad the technique is working.

INNOCENT: Yes.

NICHOLAS: Excellent.

INNOCENT: Yes. When I do this nobody knows that I am talking to my voices. So they don't look at me as if I am crazy. It is normal to see people talking into their phones. Sometimes people have very intimate conversations like this. I once heard someone break up with his girlfriend on a train between Peckham Rye and Denmark Hill. Everyone was listening but nobody thought he was crazy. Except me. I would not have a conversation like that in public. Not with a real person.

NICHOLAS: So this beach holiday…

INNOCENT: Yes. My sister played all day in the sand and my mother did not have to go to work. And I played football with some other boys. They called me Michael Essien. Do you remember him?

NICHOLAS: I don't follow football.

INNOCENT: No?

NICHOLAS: No.

INNOCENT: Michael Essien was in our national team. He played for Chelsea. You don't know him?

NICHOLAS: Sorry.

INNOCENT: They called me Michael Essien because I was from Ghana too. Everyone wanted me on their team.

NICHOLAS: Do you still play football?

INNOCENT: Not any more.

NICHOLAS: Maybe it's something you should take up again.

INNOCENT: There was a pitch beside our flat. But it was not very nice there. Lots of needles. People sold drugs there.

He takes out his phone again and answers it.

Please go away now. I have told you I cannot speak to you at this moment. I am talking to my psychiatrist and it is very important that I listen to him. Thank you.

He puts his phone away.

Pause.

NICHOLAS: Well, Innocent, you've made a lot of progress.

INNOCENT: Perhaps I can stop the medication?

NICHOLAS: I don't think we should rush anything.

INNOCENT: It makes me very sleepy.

NICHOLAS: Yes. But it is also helping with your recovery. But I'm very pleased that some of the techniques that we have taught you here are also working. Things are looking very positive. You'll be able to go home very soon.

INNOCENT: Yes, I think so too. Maybe I will start to play football again.

NICHOLAS is drinking.

GRACE: So what does that mean?

NICHOLAS: They call it a serious untoward incident and there'll be an inquiry.

GRACE: But you've had people commit suicide before.

NICHOLAS: The family are saying the hospital was negligent. Apparently her girlfriend kept phoning the crisis team because she was getting very stressed. But the message didn't get passed on – they were understaffed.

GRACE: Well that's not your fault.

NICHOLAS: It wouldn't have happened if I hadn't been off sick.

He drinks.

Bloody ATOS.

GRACE: What?

NICHOLAS: They did an assessment and they said she was fit for work so her benefit got cut and she had to go back to cleaning.

GRACE: Well there you are!

He drinks.

What was it about Janet?

NICHOLAS: What?

GRACE: You talked about her a lot.

NICHOLAS: No more than you talk about Dorothy Grainger.

GRACE: You always say it's not good to get too attached to patients.

NICHOLAS: The woman's just committed suicide Grace.

GRACE: I'm sorry.

NICHOLAS: It's just one thing after another with this fucking job. You have to be a mug to do it. There's me with damp patches on the wall of my office and there's fucking Graham Lloyd OBE with his spanking new private hospital and his patients that adulate him.

GRACE: Don't start that again, Nick.

NICHOLAS: At Oxford I used to laugh at friends like Graham who were so focused on money and success. Turns out he's the saviour of the world! Going off to climb Kilimanjaro to raise money for cancer research with his new young wife.

GRACE: Is that what you want, a new young wife?

NICHOLAS: Don't be ridiculous.

GRACE: How old was Janet?

NICHOLAS: About your age.

She takes this in.

You know, fifty looms and all you can see ahead is a gradual decline of your mental powers and you realize that you should have forged ahead when you were in your twenties like all those arrogant bastards you were at University with. They were right all along. And you've missed the fucking boat.

GRACE: Nick, stop it!

NICHOLAS: What?

61

GRACE: Just stop it.

NICHOLAS: Is that what you say to Dorothy Grainger when she moans about being lonely?

GRACE: I'm her priest. It's my job to listen to her. Which I do. Just like you listen to your patients. But then I come home to you and I'm expected to listen to you lacerating yourself like this night after night. And if I say anything, you dismiss it and start treating me as if it's somehow my fault. I can't bear it Nick! It's unbearable. Lying beside you every night in that bed feeling guilty that I can't solve it for you. If the job makes you that unhappy then do something else.

NICHOLAS: Oh there's a vote of confidence in my abilities!

GRACE: Get some help Nick. For both our sakes.

The Beach. It's raining.

PATRICK: I'm not going back.

NICHOLAS: Dad. You're getting soaked.

PATRICK: Bit of rain never hurt anyone.

NICHOLAS: At least put your mac on.

PATRICK: I don't need a mac. She wants to get me put in some institution.

NICHOLAS: No-one's going to put you anywhere. She just wants you to have some tests.

PATRICK: Why can't you all leave me alone? You doctors you're all the same.

NICHOLAS: You're a doctor.

PATRICK: Mmmm?

Pause. He sits in the sand. Starts digging with an abandoned plastic spade.

NICHOLAS: Dad.

PATRICK: Oh Nick. When did you come?

NICHOLAS: I came for lunch. We had lunch together.

PATRICK: Ah.

He looks at Nick.

I'm having a bad day, aren't I?

NICHOLAS: Yes, I think you are.

PATRICK: Some days are worse than others.

NICHOLAS: Yes.

PATRICK: Your mother is very worried about you.

NICHOLAS: About me?

PATRICK: This patient of yours who committed suicide.

NICHOLAS: She shouldn't have told you about that.

PATRICK: Why not?

NICHOLAS: It's nothing to worry about.

PATRICK: Is there going to be a coroner's inquiry?

NICHOLAS: Yes.

PATRICK: Discharge her too early did you?

NICHOLAS: Why do you say that?

PATRICK: You were always jumping the gun.

NICHOLAS: It's what I do. What I've been trained to do.
Judge whether someone is a danger to themselves or other
people, assess their state of mind, discharge them if I think
they're fit to come off section.

PATRICK: Bloody doctors.

NICHOLAS: Mmmm?

PATRICK: Eh? And was she?

NICHOLAS: What?

PATRICK: Fit to be discharged?

NICHOLAS: I thought so. But my ward manager is saying she
should have been put on a depot first. Look, why don't we
go back up to the house.

PATRICK: Why wasn't she put on a depot?

NICHOLAS: I didn't think she needed it.

PATRICK: But you thought wrong?

NICHOLAS: She had a relapse.

PATRICK: You should have foreseen that lad.

NICHOLAS: Unlike you Dad, I'm not omniscient.

PATRICK: I kept my eye on the ball. I was an oncologist.

NICHOLAS: I know.

Seagulls.

PATRICK: Seagles.

NICHOLAS: What?

PATRICK: I used to bring my son here for our holidays.

NICHOLAS: Did you?

PATRICK: He's a psychiatrist. Very clever.

NICHOLAS: Really?

PATRICK: Yes. I'm very proud of him. Sensitive lad. Always was. Bit of a bleeding heart. But damned clever. Got a First at Oxford. Wants to save the world. Ha!

NICHOLAS watches him play in the sand with the spade.

HOPE, INNOCENT AND NICHOLAS

HOPE and INNOCENT are waiting for NICHOLAS.

INNOCENT: Doctor Hamilton said I will be able to come home very soon. I'll be there for Precious's birthday.

HOPE: You must be sure you are well first. Last time they let you out a little soon.

INNOCENT: Don't you want me at home?

HOPE: Of course I want you at home.

Pause.

Your father wants us to go out there for her birthday. Precious has never been to Ghana. He has sent money for the tickets.

INNOCENT: When are we going to go?

HOPE: I have to make sure I can get the time off work.

INNOCENT: Will we be staying with Nana?

HOPE: Maybe.

INNOCENT: I miss Nana.

NICHOLAS enters.

NICHOLAS: Ah, sorry. Yes. Thanks for coming up, Mrs. Asamoah. How are you today, Innocent?

INNOCENT: I'm good.

NICHOLAS: Grand. Well. The good news is that we think you've made great progress. We're all very hopeful.

INNOCENT: So can I go?

HOPE: Listen to the doctor, Innocent.

INNOCENT: We are going to Ghana for my sister's birthday.

NICHOLAS: *(Looking at HOPE.)* Ah?

INNOCENT: It is her fourteenth birthday and we are going back to Ghana to stay with my grandmother.

NICHOLAS: Right. When is this?

HOPE: I am taking Precious to see her father.

NICHOLAS: When?

HOPE: We leave next week.

INNOCENT looks at her.

NICHOLAS: So…?

HOPE: But Innocent's aunty and uncle will be visiting him.

NICHOLAS: Oh I see. So Innocent isn't actually going?

HOPE looks at INNOCENT.

HOPE: Do you think he is well enough, Doctor?

INNOCENT looks at NICHOLAS.

NICHOLAS: We need to think very carefully about discharging you, Innocent. We're worried that you won't take your medication.

INNOCENT: You said I was making progress.

NICHOLAS: You undoubtedly are but there are a lot of factors we have to take into consideration. We need to know that you are going to be compliant. It's important that you carry on with the olanzapine.

INNOCENT: I'm not going to hurt anyone.

NICHOLAS: I'm sure you're not.

INNOCENT: And I'm not going to kill myself.

NICHOLAS: We think you need to accept your status as a patient with a serious illness.

INNOCENT: You said I was better.

HOPE: The doctor knows best, Innocent.

INNOCENT looks at her.

INNOCENT: This is him, isn't it?

HOPE: Who?

INNOCENT: My father. He doesn't want me there.

HOPE: Please Innocent.

NICHOLAS: I'm sure your family's first concern is that you get yourself completely well.

INNOCENT: I am well. But if I have to stay in here I will become sick again.

NICHOLAS: You might think you're well but we are better placed than you to make that judgement.

INNOCENT: Did he send the money for my ticket?

HOPE: Not now Innocent.

INNOCENT: He didn't, did he? He's ashamed of me.

NICHOLAS: Innocent, I promise that as soon as we think you're ready, we'll discharge you.

INNOCENT: We? Who is this "we"? I thought you were not like the rest of them.

NICHOLAS: Innocent, I'm the fucking doctor! Do you know how many years I trained to be a psychiatrist?

HOPE and INNOCENT look at him in shock.

NICHOLAS: Sorry. Sorry.

HOPE: You have upset Doctor Hamilton, Innocent.

INNOCENT: *(Defeated.)* I will miss my sister's birthday.

NICHOLAS: Maybe she can come and visit you before she goes to Ghana.

HOPE shakes her head at NICHOLAS.

Or you could speak to her on the phone. Would you like that?

INNOCENT: No-one wants to listen to me.

NICHOLAS: We think, I think you need more time.

INNOCENT goes into himself. He starts to fit as if he is drowning.

1980. NICHOLAS is in PATRICK's arms.

PATRICK: You ok?

NICHOLAS nods.

That was scary.

NICHOLAS nods.

The currents around here can be very strong.

NICHOLAS doesn't say anything.

Your Dad wouldn't let you drown.

He rubs NICHOLAS with the towel.

You know my father used to bring me here. He used to come here fishing. He had a boat he used to keep down here. My mother hated boats but he loved nothing more than to be out on the sea.

NICHOLAS: Were you a boy?

PATRICK: Yes, I was nine, ten. About your age.

NICHOLAS: Did he catch any fish?

PATRICK: Yes. We used to bring them home to my mother. But she refused to cook them. She didn't like the smell. So my father would take them out into the garden, chop their heads off and gut them and we'd make a bonfire and cook them out there in the garden under the stars.

NICHOLAS thinks about this.

Maybe we could hire a boat one day. Go out fishing. Would you like that?

NICHOLAS nods.

NICHOLAS: Would we have to eat them?

PATRICK: What else?

NICHOLAS: We could throw them back in.

PATRICK: We could. Let them live a bit longer. Is that what you'd like?

NICHOLAS nods.

NICHOLAS, JANET AND INNOCENT

JANET enters and either climbs onto NICHOLAS's back or speaks to him from behind his left shoulder.

JANET: *(Softly.)* Ooo,ooh, ahh, ahh, ahh.

NICHOLAS looks at her.

She laughs.

INNOCENT enters carrying a football. He is eating a watermelon.

He watches NICHOLAS for a while.

He holds out a piece of watermelon to him.

NICHOLAS takes it.

He eats it.

JANET: *(Softly.)* Ooo, ooo.

NICHOLAS hands some watermelon to JANET.

INNOCENT finishes his watermelon.

He starts playing with the football.

He plays keepy-uppy using his feet.

JANET and NICHOLAS continue eating their watermelon and watch.